Buddha's Guide to Healthy Eating

Mindful Nutrition for Body and Soul

Table of Contents

Chapter 1. Introduction

Dive into an enticing journey of self-discovery and well-being in our Special Report: "Buddha's Guide to Healthy Eating: Mindful Nutrition for Body and Soul". This report not only uncovers the mystical wisdom of Buddha, but also brilliantly marries it with contemporary nutritional science, creating a unique guide to achieving physical health and spiritual tranquility through food. Presented in a friendly, down-to-earth manner, this report is here to revolutionize our understanding of diet, breaking the barrier between your everyday meals and the path to inner peace. Prepare yourself to discover a world where every bite you take paves the way to better health and enhanced mindfulness. Experience this perfect blend of ancient wisdom and modern research to transform your life now, one meal at a time. It's time for a delightful and transformative read. Order your copy today. Your journey towards mindful nutrition awaits!

Chapter 2. The Art of Mindful Eating: A Buddist Perspective

Mindful eating, a habit deeply rooted in the teachings of Buddhism, is an art that many may overlook in our modern society's fast-paced lifestyle. Engaging with our food on a spiritual level extends us an invitation to experience not just the nutritional benefits of our food but ultimate emotional and spiritual nourishment as well. This practice encourages us to slow down and savor each bite, offering gratitude, focusing on the present moment, and cultivating a healthy relationship with our food.

2.1. The Principle of Mindfulness

Before immersing into the subtleties of mindful eating, it is crucial to understand the underlying principle of mindfulness. Mindfulness, in the teachings of Buddha, doesn't merely imply awareness; it involves the direction of our conscious attention without any judgement. It is the art of living in the present moment, embracing experiences as they come and depart, unembellished and pure, without the interference of past prejudices or future anxieties.

As we apply this principle to eating, we vie to be completely present during our meals, taking in the taste, smell, texture, and color of our food, savoring each bite, and offering gratitude for the nourishment it provides. Often, we eat on autopilot, our mind wandering amidst past events or future plans. Mindful eating calls us, instead, to anchor ourselves in the present, transforming each meal into not just a routine necessity, but a thoughtful meditation.

2.2. Being Present at the Table

The first notion of practicing mindful eating is being entirely present while eating. In our fast-paced lives, many of us are guilty of consuming meals in rush, distraction governing the process. It might be in front of the television, the computer, or even while cruising through tasks. This gives rise to mindless eating, which frequently leads to overeating, under-eating, or uninformed food choices–all of which can compromise our physical and psychological wellness.

Mindful eating encourages us to dedicate exclusive time for our meals. Allocate time in your day where you commit to sit down at your dining area, away from distractions, completely present with your food. Allow yourself to engage in the act of eating without juggling other tasks. Savor the taste, chew slowly, acknowledge the contribution each mouthful makes towards your well-being, providing you with energy, building materials, and support to your immune system. By being fully present, we foster a healthier and more appreciative relationship with food.

2.3. Listening to Hunger and Fullness Cues

Our body is equipped with an intrinsic wisdom that communicates its needs and limits; it signals when we're genuinely hungry and when we're satiated. Frequently, we override these signals due to emotional eating, eating out of boredom, or being disconnected from our body's needs. This often results in overeating, discomfort, guilt, and can contribute to an unhealthy relationship with food.

Through sitting quietly with ourselves, taking a few deep breaths before our meal, and consciously asking if we are indeed hungry, we can begin to listen to these signals. Simultaneously, while consuming our food, it's essential to maintain this conscious connectedness, witnessing when our body signals that we've eaten enough. Cultivating this honor for our body's wisdom can combat mindless overeating and promote a harmonious balance between our mind, body, and food.

2.4. Eating with Gratitude

In many Buddhist traditions, offering gratitude before and after a meal is a cherished ritual. By expressing gratitude, we engage in mutually beneficial act - we recognize the earth, the labor, and the lives that contributed to the meal before us, and it serves as a wonderful reminder of the interconnectedness of life.

As we offer thanks, we become more aligned with the act of eating mindfully, as gratitude activates the parasympathetic nervous system–promoting relaxation and allowing us to be fully engaged in the present moment. This act develops appreciation for our food and discourages the tendency to eat mindlessly.

2.5. Mindful Choices

Healthy eating is not just about what you eat, but how you eat it. That said, what we choose to nourish our bodies with also plays a vital role in our overall wellness, as recognized by modern nutritional science. Balance, variety, and moderation are the three pillars of a healthy diet. As mindfulness encourages awareness and conscious decision-making, it can greatly aid us in making balanced, varied, and moderate food choices.

Fostering conscious eating habits encourages us to choose foods that are nutritionally rich and corresponds to our body's needs. It discourages the consumption of food high in unhealthy fats, sugars or excessive salt. With mindful eating, our food choices become a reflection of our respect for our physical well-being.

2.6. The Spiritual Significance of Mindful Eating

Apart from the physical benefits, mindful eating also provides spiritual nourishment. By slowing down and savoring our meals, we enter a state of meditation–a pause from the rush of life. It provides an avenue to cultivate deeper self-awareness and understanding, as well as honing our capacity to reduce stress.

Mindful eating maps out the path to a more profound existential experience: that is acknowledging the interconnection of all things. As we realize the journey our food has taken to reach our plate, we appreciate the greater web of life – underlining a central theme of Buddhist philosophy.

Ultimately, the art of mindful eating is an encompassing practice that touches on physical health, emotional wellbeing, and spiritual growth. It fosters a deep connection between the mind, body, and spirit–a characteristic detail reflective of the Buddhist way of life. By consciously integrating this practice into our daily routine, we can step away from disorderly eating habits and cultivate a healthier relationship with food–one that nourishes our body and soul alike.

This wholesome practice is not about perfection, but about making small deliberate steps towards a healthier, more mindful lifestyle. Everyday holds an opportunity for growth and awareness. Each meal you sit down for is a chance to deepen your practice of mindful eating. It's an invitation to transform your relationship with food and, in essence, with your own body and life.

Chapter 3. The Interconnection of Body, Mind, and Meal

Centuries ago, beneath the shadow of the Bodhi tree, Buddha explored the irrevocable link between what we consume and who we are. Today, scientific research is giving credence to Siddhartha's epiphanies, harmonizing age-old wisdom and cutting-edge discoveries.

3.1. The Biopsychology of Eating

Understanding the physiological ramifications of our eating habits, we begin with a fundamental principle of biopsychology - the relationship between diet and brain function. Each bite we take can either fuel or starve our minds.

Under the lens of neuroscience, it's revealed that the types of food we consume can alter brain chemistry, affecting mood, cognition, and overall mental health. This process occurs through the "gut-brain axis," a communication network linking our gastrointestinal tract with the nervous system. It's through this connection that nutrients—or lack thereof—can cause ripples on the surface of consciousness.

Another essential aspect to consider is that our gut hosts about 70% of the immune system. A disturbed gut microbiome due to unhealthy eating can lead to a weakened immune response, making us more susceptible to physical as well as mental illness. This is evidence enough that there's more to mindful eating than abstract philosophical musings; it deeply impacts our health and well-being.

3.2. Eat, Feel, and Be: Decoding the Emotional Aspect

Eating is an emotionally charged experience. Traditionally, food occupies the heart of every celebration, consolation, and daily life. It demonstrates love and kind regard, and its lack can similarly evoke feelings of deprivation and sadness. Recognizing this, we can start leveraging food for emotional healing.

Jennifer Daubenmier, Ph.D., a researcher at the University of California, San Francisco, stated that "Individuals may eat high-fat, high-sugar foods in an attempt to 'self-soothe' during times of strife." By doing so, they inadvertently amplify the negative cycle, as poor nutrition further hampers emotional well-being. Instead, approaching meals mindfully can serve as a therapeutic tool, aiding emotional stability by promoting healthier food choices.

Understanding the emotional undercurrents coursing through our relationship with food creates the opportunity to chart our happiness buoyed not on the empty rewards of junk food, but on balanced nourishment.

3.3. Recipes for the Soul: Nutrition and Spirituality

Mindful eating is a meditative practice necessitating presence, gratitude, and understanding of our food sources, transforming eating into an act of spiritual growth. The Buddhist practice of non-harming or 'ahimsa' manifests in plant-first diets, reflected in the rise of vegetarianism and veganism among spiritual practitioners today.

Modern nutritional research upholds the health benefits of plant-first diets. From preventing heart disease and cancer to promoting brain health, the advantages are multifaceted. Against the backdrop of the global environmental crisis, such diets also serve as a green choice. Here, the wisdom of Buddha interweaves with scientific advice, offering a harmonious solution on a platter.

3.4. A Path to Enlightenment Through Your Plate

Building upon the spiritual-spice-infused traditions of mindful eating, remember that every meal is an open door to self-discovery. By savoring each bite, we can learn to appreciate different aspects of our meal—the color, texture, smell, and layers of flavors.

Listen to your body's signals. Develop an understanding of hunger and satiety cues. Practicing intuitive eating, paying heed to our body's needs, we can foster a healthier relationship with food—a cornerstone of well-being.

3.5. Incorporating Mindfulness into Your Everyday

Heightened awareness of the interplay of body, mind, and meal is the first step on this transformative path. So, the next time you sit down for a meal, take a moment to reflect on the bygone journey of the food and appreciate its nourishing power.

Remember, the road to mindful eating is not a simple diet switch, but a continuous journey of fostering mindfulness in every action.

As Jack Kornfield, a renowned teaching Buddhist, stated so aptly, "The trouble is, you think you have time." So, why not start today? With every meal, we have an opportunity to not just fuel our body but feed our soul and unburden the mind through the art of mindful eating, creating a harmonious melody of body, mind, and food.

In this journey of mindfulness, remember Buddha's wisdom, "To keep the body in good health is a duty... otherwise we shall not be able to keep our mind strong and clear." Let's imbibe that sense of duty in every mindful bite we take. It's time to transform your food habits, your health, and your life—one meal at a time.

Chapter 4. Decoding the Buddha Diet: A Historical Context

Regarded as one of the most enlightened beings, Buddha is known not just for his immense wisdom and spiritual teachings, but also for the unique diet he followed. An exploration into the historical context of the Buddha diet exposes an intriguing mixture of simplicity, mindfulness, and intuitive understanding of body's needs and nature's bounty.

4.1. The Simple Life

Delving into Buddha's diet begins with understanding his lifestyle. Born as Siddhartha Gautama into royal luxury, Buddha relinquished all earthly possessions in his search for enlightenment. His life, post this spiritual quest, was simple and shorn of luxury – a lifestyle that extended to his dietary habits that consisted of simple foods abundantly available in nature.

The Buddhist scriptures reference certain rules, also known as "Vinaya," governing food. The monks were allowed to eat solid food only between dawn and noon. This was not to starve or inflict difficulties upon them, but rather to mitigate any distractions so that they could focus on monastic activities. This approach advocates a form of intermittent fasting, which modern science now knows can induce autophagy, a cellular cleanup process leading to improved physical health and possibly longevity.

4.2. Mindful Eating

Equally prominent in the Buddha's eating habits was the concept of mindfulness. This involved respectful acknowledgement and conscious awareness of each morsel of food consumed. Buddha advised against eating in a hurried or absent-minded manner. Each meal was to be cherished, thoroughly masticated, and appreciated for its nourishment. Mindful eating formed an essential part of the journey towards attaining spiritual enlightenment as it brings us into the present moment, sharpening the awareness of our actions and their results on the body and mind.

Modern nutritional science has found numerous benefits to this mindful approach, including a better relationship with food, preventing overeating, aiding digestion, and improving the overall quality of life.

4.3. Nature's Bounty in the Buddha Diet

While exploring the Buddha diet, it is essential to note its foundation in natural and seasonally available foods. Buddha encouraged consumption of locally grown fruits, vegetables, and grains. By incorporating what nature readily provided, the diet was innately varied and balanced, ensuring different combinations of nutrients essential for holistic health.

Now, modern studies have shown the importance of consuming seasonal and local produce to optimise nutrient content, reduce the environmental footprint and support local agriculture.

4.4. Allergies, Intolerances, and Restrictions

Buddhist scriptures mention instances where Buddha prescribed changes to diet based on individual constitutions, reflecting an understanding of allergies and intolerances. Though primitive, this could be seen as an early instance of personalised nutrition strategy.

Taking mindful note of the body's response to different foods and excluding those causing discomfort resonates with today's personalised nutrition approach. Emerging research underscores the need for customised diets to cater to individual genetic disparities and gut microbiome variations.

4.5. The Middle Path

Perhaps the most salient feature of the Buddha's teachings, including his dietary advice, is the Middle Path. Avoiding the extremes of self-denial and self-indulgence, the Middle Path seeks a harmonious balance. The diet, too, strikes a balance between indulging the taste buds and maintaining nutritional health.

Modern nutritional science recommends a balanced approach to sustenance. Consuming a diverse range of food groups in moderation is suggested, instead of extreme diets that eliminate certain food groups entirely.

As we unravel the layers of Buddha's eating habits and dietary rules, we encounter an incredible fusion of wisdom, simplicity, and mindfulness. We find that his teachings offer a balanced and holistic perspective on nutrition, emphasizing the impact of our dietary choices on physical health and spiritual well-being.

Embodying the core tenets of Buddha's dietary philosophy into modern diets could pave the way for enhanced physical health and mental peace. As we blend the time-tested wisdom with the findings of modern nutritional science, we can chart a path to holistic well-being, nurturing both our bodies and souls.

Chapter 5. Modern Nutrition: Unwrapping the Science

Understanding the ever-evolving field of nutrition science is key to developing a healthy and sustainable eating pattern. Drawn from the latest research, this section aims to provide an in-depth exploration into modern nutrition, equipping readers with knowledge about core nutrients, their role in our well-being, and how they interact with our bodies.

5.1. The Role of Macronutrients

The human body is a complex system that continually works to maintain homeostasis — our roles in determining a resilient, healthy state. This balance heavily depends upon three principal constituents, known as macronutrients: carbohydrates, proteins, and fats.

Let's delve deeper into each of these types of macronutrients:

Carbohydrates: Often dubbed as 'energy givers', carbs are primarily used by the body to produce energy. They range from simple sugars like glucose to complex types like starch and fibers. The brain utilizes glucose, derived from carbohydrates, as its primary fuel source, making this macronutrient crucial for cognitive functions.

Proteins: Proteins are the building blocks of body tissues, like muscles and organs, and play integral roles in virtually every biological process. Made up of smaller units called amino acids, proteins are vital for cellular repair, enzymes' production, as well as strengthening the immune functions.

Fats: Once blamed for heart diseases and weight gain, fats are now understood to be essential for the body. They act as carriers for fat-soluble vitamins (A, D, E, K), constitute cell membranes, and are vital for maintaining a stable body temperature.

5.2. The Importance of Micronutrients

While macronutrients lay the foundation for our body's energy needs, micronutrients, despite being required in smaller quantities, play pivotal roles in ensuring smooth bodily functions and preventing disease. These include vitamins and minerals, each with unique benefits and necessary for diverse biological procedures.

5.3. Spotlight on Dietary Fibers

Beyond the common macros and micros, dietary fibers bring a distinctive value to the nutrition table. They aid in maintaining an effective digestive system, help control your weight, and hold a significant role in reducing the risk of diseases such as diabetes and heart disease.

5.4. Unleashing the Power of Antioxidants

Antioxidants, another vital component of nutrition, serve as bodyguards to your cells, defending against damage from harmful molecules called free radicals. They are powerful agents in battling some reputed health adversaries like heart disease, cancer, and diseases correlated to aging.

5.5. Digestion and Absorption: The Inside Story

The food we consume doesn't serve its purpose until it's properly digested and absorbed into the body. The digestive system is akin to a sophisticated factory, deconstructing food into nutrients through various stages of chemical breakdown and physical transportation.

5.6. The Impact of Processed Foods

Foods in their natural state offer the highest nutrient efficacy. Processed foods often lose their nutritional value, with manufacturers adding excessive sugars, sodium, and unhealthy fats. Becoming mindful of this fact challenges us to intentionally seek out whole, nutritious foods instead.

5.7. Interplay Between Diet and Chronic Diseases

Over 50% of adults across the globe live with a chronic condition, many of which are diet-related. Developing an understanding of how nutrition influences disease onset, progression, and management unlocks powerful tools for prevention and living a high-quality life.

5.8. Shaping Your Plate: A Balanced Approach

Putting nutritional knowledge into practice demands a personalized, balanced approach. This encompasses a diverse color palette of fruits and vegetables, lean proteins, whole grains, and healthy fat sources—Presenting the balanced plate model for a nutritious, satisfying meal.

Buddha's teachings instill balance and moderation. Incorporating these principles with modern nutritional understanding allows us to make mindful, health-enhancing dietary decisions. Evolving in our awareness of nutrition science not only contributes to physical health but deepens our connection to our bodies, cultivating respect and mindfulness for the sustenance we consume. Having garnered this enhanced understanding, we are poised at the precipice of an evolved eating pattern, advancing towards a mindful path that honours both our physical health and our spiritual tranquility.

Chapter 6. Satiety and Satisfaction: Buddha's Teachings and Eating Habits

Eating is not just a physical process; it's an integration of the body, mind, and soul. It's a profound endeavour where you nourish yourself, not only physically but also mentally and spiritually–a lesson we are about to decipher through Buddha's teachings and how it intertwines with our eating habits.

6.1. Mindful Eating: An Introduction

Mindful eating, simply put, is a practice rooted in mindfulness. Mindfulness, a principle preached extensively by Buddha, is about being completely present in the current moment.

In the context of eating, mindfulness means savouring every bite, dedicating undivided attention to the taste, texture, aroma, and even the sound of your food as you chew. Buddha stressed the importance of embracing every single moment, and through it, he embodies the art of enjoying each meal thoroughly.

Mindful eating is not restricted to the act of eating alone. It extends to recognizing the source of your food, the earth's bounty that satiates you, and acknowledging the efforts of the farmer, who toils to provide you with these fresh offerings.

6.2. Understanding Satiety

Satiety refers to a state of being satisfied or fulfilled, where the desire for further consumption is quenched. One of the key strategies to prevent overeating is understanding and listening to your hunger and satiety signals. In the context of nutrition, Buddha's teachings shed light on satiety, encouraging us to consume only as much as our body requires.

It's essential to note that satiety isn't strictly about the quantity of food consumed. It's also about the quality. Consuming nutrient-rich food versus processed and fast food will have a tremendous difference in how your body processes and perceives satiety. Through mindfulness, you learn to connect with your body's cues, enabling a much better understanding of genuine hunger versus emotional or habitual eating.

6.3. Nutritional Science and Satiety

Today's nutritional science supports Buddha's teachings on mindful eating. It emphasizes the consumption of a balanced meal comprising protein, fibre, and healthy fats–components that promote satiety.

High-fibre foods, for instance, help control the speed at which you digest your meal. This slower process means you feel fuller for longer, lessening the desire to indulge in more frequent, unnecessary snacking.

Equally, protein-rich foods also enhance feelings of satisfaction. Proteins have a more complex molecular structure, meaning your body uses more energy to metabolize them, thereby defaulting into a slower digestion rate and promoting satiety.

Healthy fats, too, have a significant role to play in boosting satiety. They prompt the release of specific hormones that signal your brain that you're full.

6.4. The Eightfold Path to Mindful Eating

Buddha's noble Eightfold Path–Right Understanding, Right Intent, Right Speech, Right Action, Right Livelihood, Right Effort, Right Mindfulness and Right Concentration–curiously, can be applied to our eating habits as well.

For instance, 'Right Understanding' implies recognizing the need for a balanced diet. 'Right Intent' involves developing a conscious intent for healthier eating habits. 'Right Speech' means speaking positively about food and body image. 'Right Action' involves placing conscious measures to improve food choices. 'Right Livelihood' advocates vegetarianism or harm-free dietary habits. 'Right Effort' is about consistent, dedicated steps towards healthy eating. 'Right Mindfulness' encourages conscious awareness of every bite. Lastly, 'Right Concentration' aids in focusing on enjoy the meal without distractions.

6.5. Blending Ancient Wisdom and Modern Science

In conclusion, Buddha's teachings and modern nutritional science share overlapping principles. Both preach mindfulness and conscious eating, promoting the sustenance of the body, while simultaneously enriching the mind and soul.

There is a growing trend towards the integration of such ancient wisdom with modern science dubbed as "lifestyle medicine." The coalescence of these dual eras of wisdom paves a much more holistic path for health and well-being, where food isn't just fuel but medicine for the body, mind, and soul.

Remember, the path to mindful eating and achieving lasting satiety doesn't happen overnight. It demands patience, commitment, and steady effort. Much like enlightenment, it's a continuous journey with its own rewards–increased awareness, appreciation for your meals, better health, and above all, inner peace.

May we all, one meal at a time, advance closer to becoming the best, healthiest version of ourselves–physically, mentally, and spiritually.

Chapter 7. The Power of Mindful Cooking: More than Just a Meal

Before taking our first steps into the world of mindful cooking, it is essential to pause and ponder what mindfulness truly means. At its core, mindfulness refers to a deep awareness of our current moment—awareness of our physical sensations, thoughts, emotions, but also an understanding of our contexts, connections, and the origins of what we consume. If we approach cooking with this mindfulness, it transforms into an arena for awareness, creativity and nourishment.

7.1. Interpreting Mindful Cooking

What then is mindful cooking? It could be defined as the practice of being fully present and engaged in the cooking process—feeling the texture of the ingredients, savoring their aromas, appreciating their colors, being aware of the noise they make while being chopped or cooked, and acknowledging the source from where they've come. As Thich Nhat Hanh, a Zen spiritual leader, puts it, "When you spend time doing your dishes—if you do them in mindfulness, you find that the dishes are not a chore, dishes are life." Similarly, the act of preparing food, if we let it, can become more than just a chore—it can turn into a nurturing practice for our body, mind, and spirit.

7.2. A Sensory Journey in the Kitchen

Engage with your senses as you cook. Let's see how:

- Observe: Begin by visually appreciating the ingredients that you are about to cook. Notice the vibrant colors, the different textures, the patterns on the surfaces. Each one is unique and beautiful in its own way.

- Touch: Feel the textures of your ingredients. The smoothness of bell peppers, the roughness of lentil grains, the rigidity of a carrot, the softness of a ripe avocado.

- Smell: Breathe in the aromas that each ingredient releases. The sweetness of caramelizing onions, the tartness of lemon, the robust aroma of fresh herbs.

- Listen: Pay attention to the sounds of your kitchen. The chop-chop of the knife, the sizzle of the pan, the whistle of the kettle, even the quiet rustling of the leaves of your salad greens.

- Taste: And finally, be aware of the flavors as you cook. Taste your dishes in different stages of cooking, understand the changes in flavor profiles.

Remember, the purpose here isn't to rush. These moments of sensory engagement provide you with an opportunity to connect more deeply with the nature and essence of food.

7.3. The Art of Conscious Ingredient Selection

Being mindful in cooking also extends to our choices of ingredients. Let's delve into some key considerations:

- Seasonal and Local: Foods that are in season and grown locally are not just fresher and tastier but also have a significantly smaller carbon footprint. Visit farmer's markets, learn and cook with what is locally available.

- Organic where possible: While not always feasible, opting for organic ingredients where you can ensures you're consuming food that's free of synthetic pesticides and additives.

- Variety and Whole Foods: Aim to incorporate a variety of both plant and animal whole foods into your meals. Not only does this offer a wealth of different nutrients, but it also keeps meals interesting and enjoyable.

- Ethically Sourced: Consider the origins of your food. Was it produced sustainably? Were the farm workers treated well? Were the animals raised in humane conditions?

7.4. Infusing Gratitude into Your Practice

While washing, cutting, and cooking, practice sending thoughts of thanks to all the people and natural elements involved in bringing these foods to your kitchen. To the sunshine, the rain, the soil, the farmer, the grocer—and the list continues. Not only does this create a deeper connection with your food, but it also brings a sense of joy and fulfillment in the process, making your culinary journey a truly spiritual one.

7.5. Mindfulness Extends Beyond the Kitchen

Lastly, mindful cooking sets the foundation for mindful eating. Savor each bite, chew slowly, and truly taste the food. Your lovingly-prepared meal deserves your full attention — not to be eaten in front of a screen or on the go.

Remember, mindful cooking isn't a skill to be mastered; it's a practice to be explored and enjoyed. So invite mindfulness into your kitchen today and begin transforming every meal into a nourishing and heartfelt experience.

As we come to conclude this chapter, it is our hope that you apply this mindfulness approach in your kitchen, carving out moments of serenity and grace amidst your daily life. Remember, every meal you prepare is a celebration of life and a profound act of love towards yourself and others. So cook with mindfulness. Cook with joy. Cook with love.

Chapter 8. The Silent Language of Food: Understanding Nutritional Symbols

Many may view food simply as sustenance, a way to satisfy hunger and provide the body with the essential nutrients it needs to function. But food, especially in the context of Buddhist philosophy and modern nutritional studies, is so much more—a vivid language of symbols waiting to reveal more profound truths about our very existence. Here, we delve into this "silent language of food," allowing it to teach us about mindfulness, well-being, and overall balance in life.

8.1. The Metaphysics of Food: Spiritual Significance and Beyond

From a Buddhist perspective, food is not just material substance—it's a dialogue between our body and our environment. Everything we eat is a product of a vast interconnected network of sentient beings, from the sunlight that falls on the plants to the farmer who cultivates the grain, imbuing our meals with much deeper significance.

This system respects all forms of life and acknowledges the simple truth that we are what we eat. Thus, an understanding of our meals is like a scaffold for an understanding of life itself. By reconnecting with the symbology of our food, we regain the ability to see this network and how we fit into it. That moment when we partake of our nourishment mindfully, we are elevating a simple, everyday act into a solemn ceremony of gratitude and interdependence.

This idea resonates well with the emerging field of nutritional psychiatry. It suggests that the quality of our food impacts not just our physical health, but our mental and emotional states as well.

8.2. Food: A Gateway to Mindfulness

The simple act of eating, when done mindfully, can become an entry point to a profound state of awareness. Even the Buddha himself held food at the center of his teachings — illustrating the pivotal role that mindful consumption plays in the attainment of spiritual tranquility.

Mindful eating is a practice rooted in the philosophy of staying present in the moment. It involves paying full attention to the experience of eating and drinking both inside and 'outside' ourselves. This means noticing the colors, smells, textures, flavors, temperatures, and even the sounds when we chew our food. It takes into account where we are, how we feel, and whom we share the meal with.

Through mindful eating, we delve into a deep dialogue with our food, taking the time to relish and appreciate the dish before us, and recognize its complex journey to our plates. This acknowledgment fuels gratitude and helps us to make healthier and more sustainable food choices.

8.3. Nourishment for The Body and Soul

Modern nutritional science and the Buddhist dietary philosophy both advocate for a well-rounded, balanced diet. The main difference lies in their emphasis—while the former mainly concerns itself with physical health, the latter focuses on spiritual health.

In the realm of nutrition science, a balanced diet encompasses a variety of foods providing all essential macronutrients (proteins, fats, carbohydrates) and micronutrients (vitamins and minerals). We need these nutrients to perform a plethora of physiological functions—from supplying energy and supporting growth and development, to promoting immune function and preventing diseases.

On the other hand, Buddha's teachings outline the concept of 'ahara' or food as something that feeds not just the physical body, but our thoughts, consciousness, and emotions as well—our soul, in essence. For instance, a meal made with understanding, love, and care will nourish us deeply, whereas food prepared in anger or sadness could potentially disturb our spiritual balance.

8.4. The Impact of Diet on Our Physiology

Every morsel of food we consume has an impact on our bodies. Take, for instance, the effect of sugars on our insulin levels, or how certain fats can influence our cardiovascular health. It's a relationship well-documented by nutritional science studies.

Just as certain foods or nutrients lead to physiological health issues, they can also influence our emotional and mental well-being, highlighting a more existential relationship between us and our meal. For example, a diet high in sugar, refined carbohydrates, and processed foods can be linked to a higher risk of depression.

By understanding the energy and nutrients we gain from specific foods, and recognizing how varied diet patterns affect our physical and mental well-being, we can make more informed, mindful decisions about our dietary habits.

8.5. Mindful Nutrition: The Bridge between Health and Harmony

If we translate Buddha's wisdom into our everyday life and combine it with our understanding of modern nutritional science, we can use mindful nutrition as a bridge to bring health and harmony. Mindful nutrition may, in fact, be the most effective tool for improving your health, enhancing spiritual growth, and promoting a sense of well-being.

By focusing on the energy and impact of food and recognizing it as a language in itself, we can start to make impactful connections between what we eat and how we feel. We unleash the power to improve our mental and physical health, exploring a path to more mindful living.

Through our journey into the 'Silent Language of Food,' we see that our meals are not as silent as they may seem. With every morsel we eat, we take another step on the journey to self-awareness, peace, and harmony. It's time to listen closely to what our food is telling us, honoring its journey, and respecting the life it represents. For, in listening, we are welcoming mindfulness to our dining tables, and ultimately, into our lives.

Our daily sustenance, seen in this new light, is anything but mundane. It is a testament of our interconnectedness with the universe, a language bespeaking not just of nutrition, but most importantly, of our humanity. Together, modern nutritional science and the teachings of Buddha guide us towards a more mindful, nourishing way of eating. This holistic view of food invites us on a transformative journey delivering not just physical health but spiritual tranquility too.

Chapter 9. Balancing the Five Tastes: A Journey Through the Buddha's Plate

Throughout life, we are propelled by the rhythm of ingestion and digestion, a cycle that underpins our existence. This chapter takes you on a gratifying exploration of a particular concept central to both Buddhism and nutrition: the balance of the five tastes. Understanding and harmonizing these five essential tastes - salty, sweet, bitter, sour, and umami can bring a profound change to our perception of food and overall wellbeing.

9.1. The Essence of the Five Tastes

Each of the five tastes is associated not only with a specific flavor perceived by our tastebuds, but also with distinct nutritional contributions and influences on our body. Salty foods, often rich in minerals, maintain hydration and electrolyte balance. Sweet foods, a natural source of carbohydrates, provide us with instant energy. Bitter foods support detoxification and often contain life-saving antioxidants. Sour foods aid digestion and the absorption of minerals while foods with umami, the savory or meaty taste, are often rich in proteins and amino acids.

This staggering palette of flavors is the universe's ingenious method of guiding us to eat a balanced diet. Our taste buds, acting as discerning samplers of nutrition, can help lead us to intake the distinct amounts of nutrients necessary for our metabolism to function optimally.

9.2. The Harmonization of Tastes

Just like the Buddhist practice of the Middle Way, which seeks balance and avoids extremes, we are to harmonize these tastes on our plate and in our mouth. No single taste should predominate; each should blend harmoniously with the others, resulting in a wholesome and balanced meal.

For instance, a plate could include sweet potatoes (sweet), sprinkled with a touch of sea salt (salty), garnished with spinach (bitter), a dash of lemon juice drizzled over it (sour), and a piece of grilled mushroom (umami) on the side. This meal, simple as it is, illustrates a harmonized plate that is an amalgamation of the five principal tastes.

Striking a balance doesn't mean having all flavors in a single meal. You could consider your intake over a day or a week, introducing all five tastes in a staggered, thoughtful manner.

9.3. Mindful Eating: The Buddhist Approach

Mindful eating is a key aspect of Buddhist teaching, where the act of eating morphs into a meditation of sorts. Every morsel of food is treated with respect, every bite is savored, and each flavor is identified and recognized for its nourishing qualities. When eating becomes mindful, we realize that the natural desire for a variety of tastes is not a mere culinary indulgence but a primal instinct for balanced nutrition.

While consuming your meal, be aware of the tastes that emerge and how they make you feel. There's much to learn about yourself from your reactions to these various tastes. You might find a particular enjoyment in salty or sweet foods, or perhaps a preference for sour or bitter tastes. These preferences can reveal potential imbalances in your nutritional needs or habitual consumption tendencies to fulfill emotional needs.

9.4. Nurturing Balance, Nourishing the Soul

Understanding and integrating the Buddha's philosophy of the five tastes introduce a new perspective to our existing eating habits. It's not just about overhauling a diet but altering our approach to food.

Much like the cycles of life, our meals should not be stagnant and unvaried. Tastes are seasonal by nature. Different vegetables and fruits available throughout the year offer different notes of tastes. A mindful eater adapts his plate accordingly, aligning the food rhythm with the rhythm of nature.

Eating by this philosophy allows the balance of five tastes not only on our plate but also in our life. Each taste contributes uniquely towards the body's wellness, supporting different organs, promoting various nutrients, and overall, nurturing an equilibrium of health.

9.5. The Journey Forward

We urge you to imbibe this wisdom of balancing the five tastes, thereby transforming the act of merely eating into a mode of self-nurturing. Keep this knowledge close when you're arranging your plate and nourishing your body. Remember, it's not about perfection but progress.

Recognize that this is a journey where the destination is not as important as the path itself - a journey of learning, unlearning and constant growth. It's a commitment to prosperity; prosperity of health, tranquility, and the utmost respect for food and life.

The path to wellbeing, as Buddha teaches, lies not in seeking new landscapes, but in having new eyes. These 'new eyes' are here within this chapter's teaching. Incorporate these lessons bit by bit into your culinary routine and relish the journey of your dynamic adjustment towards a mindful, balanced diet. Your pursuit of health and tranquility awaits one harmonious plate at a time.

Chapter 10. Transformative Recipes: Wholesome Dishes, Wholesome Life

Eating mindfully, as taught by Buddha, is not just about what you eat but also how you eat. In this chapter, we're incorporating spiritual wisdom with modern nutritional science. The following recipes that we'll delve into are designed to not only feed your body but nourish your mind and soul. With an array of flavors and nutritional benefits, all these delicacies are both good for your health and inviting for your taste buds. Let's start this sumptuous journey!

10.1. Mindful Eating: The Basis

The art of mindful eating is deeply rooted in the beliefs of Buddha. For him, meals were not merely a means to quench hunger, but instead, they were an act of meditation, an opportunity to connect with ourselves, our environment, and our food. When you eat mindfully, every bite you take becomes an experience of joy and gratitude.

But what does this mean in practical terms? Mindful eating is all about:

- Taking the time to eat and giving your full attention to your meal.

- Experiencing the flavors, smells, sounds, textures, and colors of your food.

- Acknowledging the complex journey the food has taken from the soil to your plate.

- Eating in a calm environment where you feel relaxed and at peace.

- Not eating too much or too little, but just enough to nourish yourself without causing discomfort or distress.

Integrating mindful eating into your daily routine is transformative. And it starts on your plate. The forthcoming section presents recipes that enable you to do just that.

10.2. Buddha Bowls: Harmony in A Bowl

Buddha bowls, named after their round Buddha belly-like shape, are all about balance and diversity. Known for their colorfulness and nutritional completeness, they often consist of a grain, a protein, lots of vegetables, a healthy fat, and a flavorful dressing.

To create your own Buddha bowl, follow the guidelines below:

Grains: Start with a base of wholesome carbohydrates. Try whole grains like brown rice, quinoa, or farro. Aim for a portion that makes up about a quarter of your bowl. These will provide you with energy and essential nutrients.

Protein: Choose from lean proteins like tofu, tempeh, chickpeas, lentils, or, if you're not vegetarian, try grilled chicken or fish. All these options are filled with essential amino acids your body needs to function.

Vegetables: Fill half your bowl with an array of colorful vegetables in an effort to benefit from different types of nutrients. Consider roasted sweet potatoes, spiralized zucchini, steamed broccoli, or fresh salad greens.

Healthy fats: Add avocados, olives, nuts or seeds to ensure you're getting the essential fatty acids that help keep you satiated.

Dressing: A flavorful dressing can elevate your Buddha bowl.

Experiment with different combinations like tahini-lemon, ginger-soy, or peanut-lime dressings.

Creating a Buddha bowl is less about strictly following a recipe and more about applying mindful eating principles. Tailor your bowl according to your personal preferences, nutritional needs, and seasonal availability of ingredients.

10.3. Mindful Curry: Comfort with Complexity

Curry is usually associated with taste-bud-tantalizing flavors and healthy ingredients. Here's a simple but robust curry recipe that engages all senses:

For the curry paste, you will need garlic, ginger, turmeric, chili, lemongrass, and coriander. Blend these ingredients with a little water until they form a paste. Sauté the paste in a little bit of coconut oil until it's aromatic, then add in chopped veggies of your choice. Add coconut milk and simmer until the vegetables are tender.

As the curry simmers, take a moment to appreciate the aroma of the simmering spices. When you serve it, observe its rich color and taste it thoughtfully, paying attention to the intricate flavors and textures it offers.

10.4. Fruits of Enlightenment: Sweet Treats

While Buddha encouraged a simple and restrained lifestyle, balance is also key to the path of enlightenment. And that includes the occasional sweet treat prepared with wholesome ingredients. Fruits and natural sweeteners can create satisfying desserts that are also nutritious.

For a simple, mindful dessert, try grilled bananas with a sprinkling of cinnamon, served over Greek yogurt and a drizzle of honey. Notice the juxtaposition of hot and cold, sweet and tangy, as you savor each component of the dessert.

By preparing and savoring these recipes, you're connecting with the principles of mindful eating, promoting physical health, and cultivating spiritual well-being. Remember, the art of mindful eating is about much more than simple nourishment! Breaking bread is a spiritual act that allows us to connect with the world around us and our inner selves. Make every meal a mindfulness experience and observe the transformative effects this practice has on your life.

Chapter 11. Continuity and Change: Applying Buddha's Teachings to Everyday Life

The Buddha's teachings aren't just about living a life of mindfulness and introspection, they also delve into how one should nourish their physical vessel - the body. Observe the natural flow of life and our regular eating habits. The continual process of nourishing your body and nurturing your mind happen in congruence - a correspondence that can lead to enlightenment about our whole selves. By integrating Buddha's teachings with a mindful approach to eating, we construct a springboard towards self-discovery, health, and inner peace.

11.1. Embrace Impermanence: Your Diet and You

Life is an endless series of changes. Our bodies change - we grow, we age. Our environments change - seasons shift, ecosystems adapt. And correspondingly, our dietary needs transform. The Buddha taught that nothing is permanent and everything is subject to change. This concept of impermanence (anicca in Pali) is key in approaching how we eat.

Understanding and accepting the concept of impermanence lead to flexibility in our diets. Rigid dietary dogmas or the latest fads don't fit into a mindful, Buddha-inspired approach to nutrition. Instead, eating becomes an intuitive process, guided by listening to what your body needs in a given moment. We must understand that our dietary needs may vary according to our age, environment, activity level, and even emotional state.

11.2. Mindful Eating: A Sacred Ritual

In the rush of modern living, the act of eating becomes secondary, more of a necessity than a mindful act. We tend to eat our meals quickly, while working or watching TV. We often don't give this act the attention it deserves, overlooking the essence of eating.

Mindful eating, however, is a cornerstone Buddhist practice. The process of consuming food should not be an automatic, mindless routine, but a conscious act of nourishing your body and mind. Make every meal an occasion to slow down, focusing on the flavors, textures, and smells of your food. Appreciate those who contributed to its creation - the farmers that grew your food, the cook who prepared it, and the entire chain of life that brought it to your plate. This practice imbues a sense of gratitude, enhancing the joy of eating, and indirectly promoting better digestion.

11.3. Subsuming Self in the Community: Food and Connectedness

Once you harness mindfulness while eating, you become more connected to the food you consume and realize the interconnectedness that underpins our existence. According to Buddha, everything in this world is interconnected. Therein lies the principle of dependent origination (pratitya-samutpada) - nothing exists in isolation; everything is dependent on and influenced by many different factors.

Including this principle in our eating habits, we marvel at how food keeps us connected to the world around us. Every ingredient on your plate is a product of the Earth, the weather, the labor of farmers.

Hence, our food is a testament to our interconnectedness with nature and society. By understanding this, we foster a sense of global stewardship, inspiring us to make environmentally conscious choices, consume locally sourced food, and reduce food waste.

11.4. Moderation: The Middle Way

The Buddha's path, referred to as the 'Middle Way,' advocates for moderation in all aspects of life - including food. By avoiding the two extremes of self-indulgence and self-denial, we find balance and harmony. Overeating can lead to a myriad of health problems, while malnutrition can leave us weak and susceptible to diseases.

Practicing moderation fosters a healthy relationship with food. It propels us to eat to nourish ourselves, rather than for mere pleasure or out of boredom. Maintaining a balanced diet, rich in a variety of foods, provides us with essential nutrients without showing favoritism to particular meals or food groups over others.

11.5. Bodily Autonomy: Choose What's Right for You

Each one of us is unique, as are our dietary needs and preferences. Applying Buddha's teachings to our diets isn't about adhering to strict dietary rules. Rather, it's about cultivating self-awareness, learning to listen to our bodies, and understanding our needs.

Buddha stressed the importance of individual autonomy by advising his followers to believe nothing until they have personally tested and experienced it. Emulate this in your pursuit of a healthy diet. Experiment with different foods and dietary patterns until you find what works best for you.

11.6. Irrevocably Intertwined: Physical Well-being & Spiritual Tranquility

Physical health and mental well-being are irrevocably intertwined. You cannot achieve complete wellbeing if you only address one aspect alone. The Buddha's teachings reflect the same - deeply recognizing the connection between the body and the mind.

Approaching your diet through the lens of Buddhist philosophy does not only promise physical well-being, but it also has profound implications for spiritual tranquility. Eating mindfully and healthily can indeed be a powerful vehicle for self-improvement and self-discovery.

In conclusion, Buddha's teachings offer a remarkable perspective on our dietary habits. By practicing mindful eating, abiding by the Middle Way, acknowledging our individual needs, and embracing change - we can build a profound relationship with food. This approach doesn't just contribute to healthier bodies, but also helps cultivate a more peaceful, mindful, and interconnected existence.

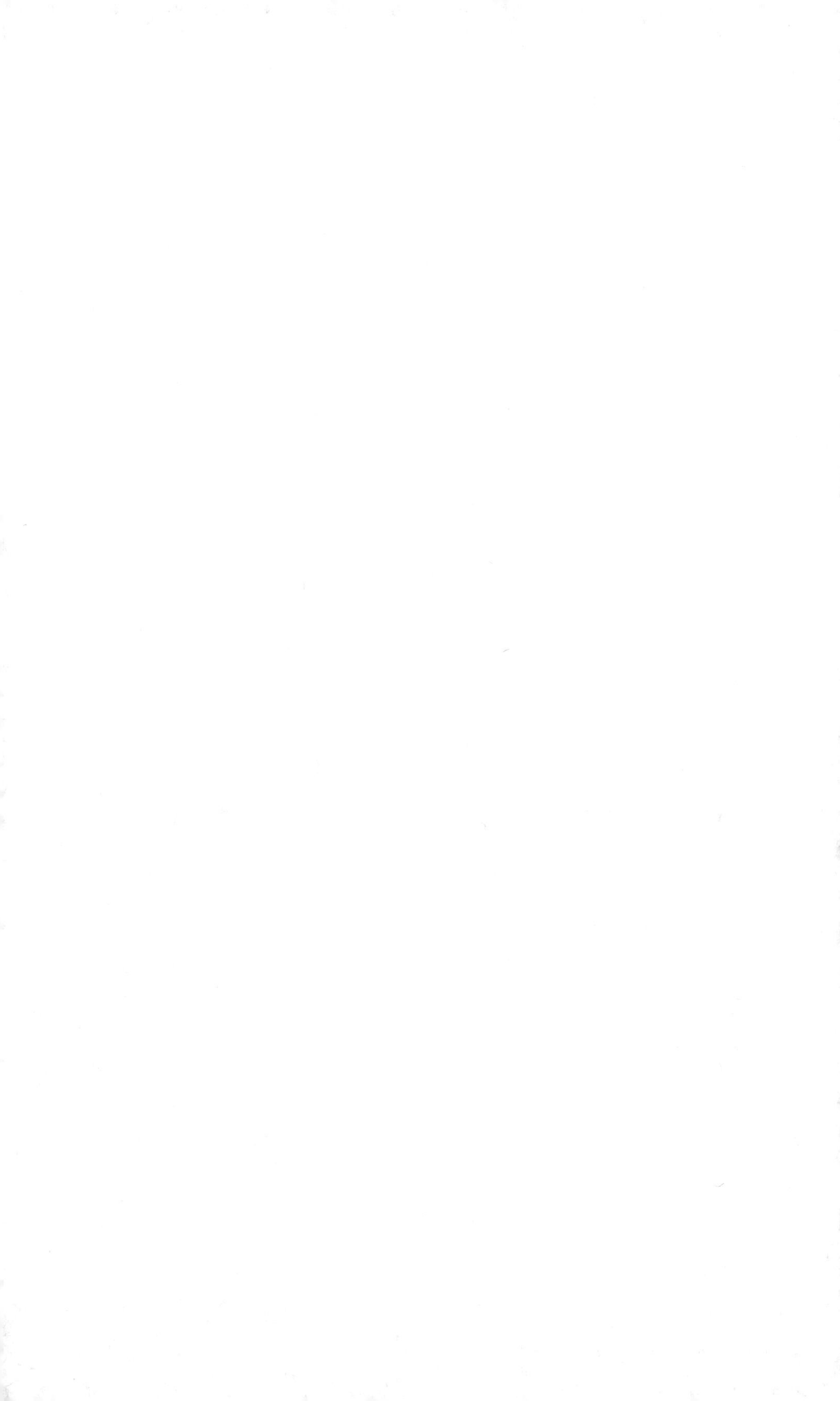